Turning 65

Kimmy Gerred

©Copyright 2018

Nelson Publishing Solutions

All Rights Reserved Copyright © 2018

By Nelson Publishing Solutions All rights reserved.

This book or any portion thereof may not be reproduced or used in any manner whatsoever without the express written permission of the publisher except for the use of brief quotations in a book review.

Printed in the United States of America First Printing, October 2018 Nelson Publishing Solutions 392 E. Stevens Rd. G13 Palm Springs, CA. 92262

Find more resources

At https://cainsure.blogspot.com

Or at www.cahealthinsure.blogspot.com

Also, find Kimmy On Facebook at
https://www.facebook.com/InsureCalifornia/

In Dedication to

Mother Nell Summers

Mother Nell was my best friend for over ten years. She was a prophet of God who sowed great spiritual stamina into my life. She became more than a mother to me. I miss her still to this day and she has been gone over ten years now.

Mother Nell held prayer meetings at her home on Woodridge road in Jackson, MS. for over 50 years. She dedicated her life in service to the Lord. She said that she was Heaven's reporter.

When 911 happened, she was in her late eighties. I asked her (because I love to glean the wisdom of our seniors as they are some of the wisest people in the earth) "Mother Nell, do you think we should go to war?" She replied "Kimi, I don't think we have a choice" and she went on to tell me that God spoke through a bush once and HE is speaking through a Bush once more.

She also said that President Bush knew some other things that we did not know about what happened on 911. And she said that "God was overturning the money changing tables" concerning 911.

I've prayed and sought to replace her presence in my life but that has not happened and I doubt that it ever will. This should be a lesson to all to cherish the people and relationships that mean something to you.

An Aging Society

Abstract

Purpose: To determine the results of a community educational structure developed to increase social activity, reduce stress and reduce loneliness while teaching skills that enhance life behavioral health skills.

Methods: A sect of elderly population were gathered into specific categories by ethnicity, finances, and education then tested and taught the 4 month "CAN" program skills. Results compared and evaluated.

Results: Significant improvements between different sects of the groups. Particular improvements of social activity were noted amongst ethnic groups with low income and ethnic groups with higher education.

Conclusion: Teaching the 16 week life skills program of "CAN" resulted in much benefited health for senior citizens providing a higher quality of life for the participants.

Key Words and Tags: Prevention Research, Elderly, Loneliness, Aging, Senior Citizens, CAN, Community Based Education, ANOVA, Perceived Stress Scale, Mastery Scale, Loneliness Scale

Program and Purpose

"CAN" is a four-month program broken down into 15 lessons with pretest and post-tests given to help evaluate the results. The program was implemented at 20 sites in rural and urban (American Journal of Health Promotion areas of Nevada in the county of Clark between 1999 and 2004 (Collins & Benedict, p. 46, 2006). The 15 lessons are taught in a 16-week period and teach the following;

1. Personal Safety (such as reducing accidents at home)

2. Financial strategies to manage limited resources

3. General wellness (such as immunizations and hand washing)

4. Productive aging

Along with encouraging wellness education that "relates instruction to practice. Lifelong learning, physical activity, social support, moderate drinking, and less smoking promote healthy aging."

"CAN" was developed to research the effects of a supportive community-based health program built to help seniors reduce stress and loneliness that teaches them skills to develop mastery on healthy aging. ANOVA, The UCLA Loneliness Scale, PSS and The Mastery Scale were used to measure the data (Collins & Benedict, p. 46, 2006).

Setting and Participants

"CAN" was provided to select number of 339 that was divided into different groups of seniors using "ANOVA (2X3X4). Each group is formed by ethnicity, education and income." The "CAN" program took place in 20 different communities throughout Nevada in Clark County. And the pretest and post-test were self-administered.

Then there were sub groups for ethnicity into Caucasian and ethnic minorities, then "by income to three different levels ($0 to $9,999; $10,000$19,999; and $20,000 or more)" and lastly, "by education to four levels (not completed high school; high school graduate; some college/ college degree; and graduate work/graduate degree." (Collins & Benedict, p. 46, 2006).

80% of the group were female so they didn't separate by gender.

Data was retained for this analysis from 36 seniors "Can" sessions.

Major Health Issues Addressed

"Loneliness has been shown to have a negative impact on health outcomes, including increased mortality, diminished recovery from illness, and a greater health service utilization, such as nursing home admission.

The ability to cope effectively with stress is seen in older adults with strong social support systems more than in their lonelier peers. Stress, or the degree to which participants perceive their recent daily life to be uncontrollable or unpredictable, would be a negative indicator of mastery." (Collins & Benedict, p. 45, 2006).

The main goal of "CAN" was to reduce stress and loneliness for senior citizens. They approached this by teaching personal safety and financial management skills.

An important skill that they taught was hand washing. They didn't mention teaching daily dental hygiene or food expiration checks importance for refrigerated foods in this article.

Results

They found that there was more social activity among the groups of ethnic minorities with lower incomes and ethnic higher education.

Overall, they found that Community Supported Health Education increases the promotion of healthy aging. Interactive educational enhancement seems to transform healthier aging by rewarding the participants with ongoing learning and practical daily achievements towards mastery. (Collins & Benedict, p. 48, 2006).

"An important finding of this study is that whereas participants showed statistically significant improvements in mastery, loneliness, and stress measures, minority participants with low incomes and those with formal educational levels showed the greatest reduction impact on those at higher risk of health problems. Such findings raise questions regarding how this occurs and whether such impacts last over time, warranting further investigation into such issues." (Collins & Benedict, p. 48, 2006).

Contributions and Studies Useful Contributions

ANOVA, The UCLA Loneliness Scale, PSS and The Mastery Scale were all part of the contributions. The seven item Mastery Scale was contributed by Pearlin and Schooler, The UCLA Loneliness Scale and the Perceived Stress Scale (PSS-10) were also contributions.

The study itself was a useful contribution to help healthcare facilities around the world know how to better care for and help the elderly have a healthy aging process.

Resources:
Grembowski D, Patrick D, Diehr P, et al. Selfefficacy and health behavior among older adults. J
Health Soc Behav. 1993; 34:89-104

Krause N, Herzog AR, Baker E. Providing support to others and well-being in late life. J Gerontol B Pyschol Sci. 1992; 47:300-311

Find more resources

At https://cainsure.blogspot.com

Or at www.cahealthinsure.blogspot.com

Also, find Kimmy On Facebook at
https://www.facebook.com/InsureCalifornia/

How Well Do We Care For Our Seniors?

What I find most important from the studies of the "CAN" program is that seniors who are more socially connected to friends and family remain healthier longer and are able to recover from health setbacks better than their companions who are more lonely or isolated. I believe this information is vital and pertinent to all ages of our society not just the elderly. (Collins & Benedict, p. 48, 2006)

The elderly are more vulnerable if they are the ones who are left alone or isolated without any true friends or family. Because they are in a much frailer condition to begin with. Sadly, it is the elderly who are the most lonely and isolated people in our society.

The scripture says in James 1:27 (KJV) "Pure religion, undefiled before God and the Father, is this: to visit the fatherless and widows in their affliction, and to keep himself unspotted from the world."

And many times they are unable to clean as well as they could when they were younger. Or they may not be able to see as well as they once could, so they might not be able to cook as well and they may not even drive anymore. So the friends, companions and family members should offer to drive them for their weekly errands and to take them a plate of cookies or a hot meal sometime.

In the third chapter of First John we are instructed how to care for those who are needy in our community. "But whoso hath this world's goods and seeth his brother have need, and shutteth up the compassion of his heart from him, how dwelleth the love of God in him? 1 John 3:17

Next, we will be evaluating some very helpful websites that can reduce stress off of our senior citizens and their care givers. You can find the website address and rating on the evaluation forms too. We are including this for your convenience.

Aging Care Website Evaluation

Website URL: http://www.agingcare.com/

Website title: Aging Care

On a scale of 1–10, with 10 being highest, rank the following:

___10__1. Is the design of the site pleasant to view?

___10__2. Is the site designed so that it is efficient for you to navigate?

___10__3. Is the site designed so that an elderly person could navigate it?

___10__4. Is the content of the site easy to understand?

___10__5. Is the content of the site factual?

___10__ 6. Would the content of the site be helpful to an aging person?

___10__ 7. Can you tell who is responsible for the authorship of the site? If so, who?

___10__ 8. Does it seem as though the authors are credible? Why or why not?

___10__ 9. Are links available to other sites? If so, are they working links to reliable sites?

___10__ 10. Overall impression

Total score (out of 100): ____100_____

The Aging Care website has many different services offered to help seniors have easy accessible contacts and information that every senior will need at some point in their transition to the retiring age. Services such as Caregiver support, Senior Living, Elder Care, Money and Legal. Also, senior medical staff who support the website.

What I like most of all about this site is that it has an active ongoing blog for new information and updates and it is visible on the front page of the website. One of the main articles that I found on the website that is impeccable for vital information is this one with ten government organizations listed that is imperative information for seniors to have easy access to such as Social Security and Medicare.

The url for that article listed on this website is as follows: http://www.agingcare.com/Articles/10Government-Programs-Caregivers-Can-Accessfor-Their-Elderly-Parents-120513.htm

This is one of the most useful websites that a senior will find on the internet and it is very easy to use. Links and tabs are clearly visible and do not over crowd the front page while providing vital information on the front page as well as all of the other pages. It even includes information about pharmaceutical programs.

Medicare Website Evaluation

Website URL https://mymedicare.gov/

Website title: Medicare.Gov

On a scale of 1–10, with 10 being highest, rank the following:

___10___ 1. Is the design of the site pleasant to view?

___10___ 2. Is the site designed so that it is efficient for you to navigate?

___10___ 3. Is the site designed so that an elderly person could navigate it?

___10___ 4. Is the content of the site easy to understand?

___10___ 5. Is the content of the site factual?

___10___ 6. Would the content of the site be helpful to an aging person?

__10__ 7. Can you tell who is responsible for the authorship of the site? If so, who?

__10__ 8. Does it seem as though the authors are credible? Why or why not?

__10__ 9. Are links available to other sites? If so, are they working links to reliable sites?

__10__ 10. Overall impression

Total score (out of 100): ____100____

The Medicare website has many different services offered to help seniors have easy accessible contacts and information that every senior will need at some point in their transition to the retiring age. Services such as Medicare Coverage,

Medicare Costs, Sign up for Medicare, Change Medicare Plan, Drug Coverage (Part D), Supplements & Other Insurance, Claims & Appeals, Manage Your Health, Forms Help & Resources. Also, the website is interactive so that it lets you submit information right from the Medicare.gov website.

Medicare.gov allows users to choose a "username" and log in when they go to the website so that the vital information is protected and an online file is opened for them to make it easier for their information to be stored and recalled when needed.

They have easy to use interactive submit buttons for seniors to add their user names and passwords and a guided tour interactive button in case they need or want extra help. They also have a "LIVE" chat compatibility to make it easier for them to get help without using a phone or postal mail. They also have interactive tabs to do research on the different plans of Medicare that they are interested in. And there is contact information available for them to reach the Medicare.gov if they have any further questions. There is also special help and care providers for seniors suffering from kidney disease and the list provides nursing homes, dialysis centers and hospitals.

The url for the interactive submit buttons for the local area contact information can be found here: : http://www.medicare.gov/your-medicarecosts/part-a-costs/part-a-costs.html

This is one of the most useful websites that a senior will find on the internet and it is very easy to use. Links and tabs are visible and on the front page while providing vital information on the front page as well as all of the other pages. It even includes information about pharmaceutical drug coverages.

Arthritis Foundation Website Evaluation

Your name: Kimmy Gerred

Website URL: http://www.arthritis.org/

Website title: Arthritis Foundation

On a scale of 1–10, with 10 being highest, rank the following:

_10___ 1. Is the design of the site pleasant to view?

_10___ 2. Is the site designed so that it is efficient for you to navigate?

_10___ 3. Is the site designed so that an elderly person could navigate it?

_10___ 4. Is the content of the site easy to understand?

_10___ 5. Is the content of the site factual?

_10___ 6. Would the content of the site be helpful to an aging person?

_10___ 7. Can you tell who is responsible for the authorship of the site? If so, who?

_10___ 8. Does it seem as though the authors are credible? Why or why not?

_10___ 9. Are links available to other sites? If so, are they working links to reliable sites?

_10___ 10. Overall impression

Total score (out of 100): __100__

The Arthritis Foundation provides information about the many types of arthritis and ways to combat it. Including ways to get involved in becoming an advocate of support for patients, constituents and family members suffering from the painful effects of this debilitating and life challenging illness.

They also provide information on self-help exercise classes throughout the nation that people can join or get involved with to help them recover or deal with the effects of this painful health condition.

There are helpful phone number contacts and addresses and internet email contacts provided so that seniors can reach out and contact the arthritis foundation, support groups, advocate volunteer sign ups, or even the exercise programs. The contact information is easy to find on the front page.

There is even an interactive submit button for them to find local offices by adding their own zip code into the website search engine to bring up all the local help provided nearby where they live.

They will find help for degenerative disk disease, rheumatoid arthritis, osteoarthritis, tendonitis, bursitis and many other arthritis related issues.   And links and information how to master living with arthritis effectively.

Personal Interviews of the Elderly

Kimmy Gerred

Abstract:

Interviews Purpose: To get a better understanding of the mind frame of elders within three different age categories from (65-74, 75-84, 85+) of nine specific areas and questions relating to their life.

Interviews Methods: Data, answers and information were collected from nine exact questions given to each person within their age.

Interviews Results and Personal Reflections: Answers varied widely but all had expectations and hopes for the future. Some appeared more reasonable and achievable than others.

Interviews Conclusion and Perceptions of Aging: We should never assume that a person quits living, hoping or dreaming regardless of their age.

We should continue to help people retain their independence. And we should continue to try and make life easier for those with mobility challenges and cognitive changes that are associated with aging.

Key Words and Tags: Prevention Research, Elderly, Loneliness, Aging, Senior Citizens

Personal Interviews

Interview of an elderly person age 65-74 years of age

Dr. HJP (Pseudonym)

Question 1. What is your age?

Dr. HJP is 70 years old. He was born in Austria. He studied at California State University and in Austria.

Question 2. Looking back over your life what is one thing that makes you proud;

Because he was a professor of Science and he just finished writing a couple of books. And he is a

Kumbha a very ingenious and intuitive. He is volatile and lively. He is quarrelsome with an aversion to indifference. He is a reformer, he is also an innovator and intellectual.

Question 3. What is your future goal?

Build a Fusion Power plant and magnetic generator and magnetic motor project.

Question 4. If you could give advice to the younger generation what would it be?

Educate yourself. Education is the key to longevity. And enjoy your life. Don't get stressed.

Question 5. What is the major change you've seen in our world in your lifetime and has it been a good one or a bad one?

Too many wars. And it was a bad change in our world.

Question 6. Is there anything you would do differently if you had it to do over again? No.

Question 7. What is the major challenge that you are facing now that you didn't have to deal with when you were younger?

To change some of the energy technology from the negative to the positive aspects of operations. And work on his lower back problems.

Question 8. What is the one thing you enjoy doing?

Working and keeping active in his favorite hobbies. Favorite hobbies; singing, swimming, scuba diving

Question 9. What is the one thing that I didn't ask you about that you want to tell me or want the other students to know? He is a good singer and he has traveled very extensively.

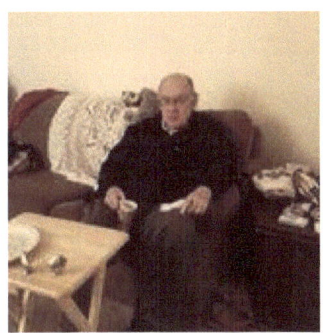

Interview of an elderly person age 65-74 years of age

Mr. Sachs 5th Blvd. (Pseudonym)

Question 1. Age

Mr. Sachs 5th Blvd is 70 years old going on two

Question 2. As you look over your lifetime what is the one thing that makes you proud; He says it is his creativity.

Question 3. What is your future goal?

He wants to build a significant Ocean liner Maritime Museum in San Francisco, Florida or overseas.

Question 4. If you could give advice to the younger generation what would it be?

Get a broad education and look at all opportunities and make every effort to be legal.

Question 5. What is the major change you've seen in our world in your lifetime and has it been a good one or a bad one?

More information is a plus but if you are trying to accomplish something you may have too much information and get bogged down in the details and then not make a good decision.

Question 6. Is there anything you would do differently if you had it to do over again?

Yes, he would have been more attentive and helpful to his parents but he was very limited in what he could do.

Question 7. What is the major challenge that you are facing now that you didn't have to deal with when you were younger?

Financial problems that he had when he was younger continue now so that he is unable to complete the projects that he would still like to do.

Question 8.   What is the one thing you enjoy doing?

Creative projects, he loves to humor people.

Question 9.   What is the one thing that I didn't ask you about that you want to tell me or want the other students to know?

If it doesn't work one way try another. His motto is the more you encourage the more things bloom.

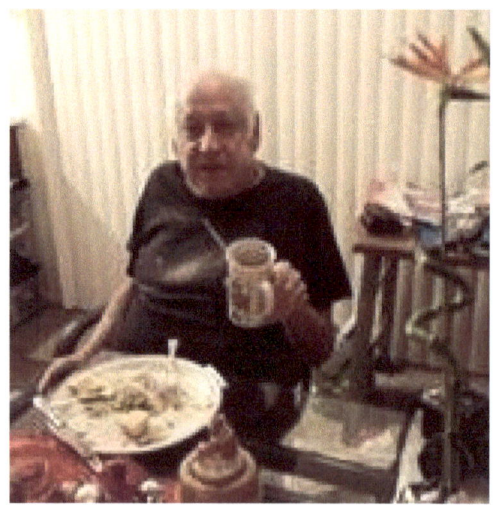

Interview of an elderly person age 75-84 year of age

Sweet Violet (Pseudonym)

Question 1. Age   81 years of age.

Question 2. As you look over your lifetime what is the one thing that makes you proud?

Her family; the ones that came before her, the ones that she bore and reared and her 23 grandchildren.

Question 3. What is your future goal?

To go to the Taj Mahal and finish her memoirs "My Life of Great Expectations" stolen from Charles Dickens "Great Expectations"

Question 4. If you could give advice to the younger generation what would it be?

Always be thankful, express gratitude, love one another and give back.

Question 5. What is the major change you've seen in our world in your lifetime and has it been a good one or a bad one?

She sees more evil around her and she feels it. And she says that it is not good.

Question 6. Is there anything you would do differently if you had it to do over again?

She would not get a divorce she would just make it through.

Question 7. What is the major challenge that you are facing now that you didn't have to deal with when you were younger?

Physical disabilities. She used to play tennis every day.

Question 8. What is the one thing you enjoy doing?

Responding to people and socializing with them.

Question 9. What is the one thing that I didn't ask you about that you want to tell me or want the other students to know? She participated in singing, dancing (Usherettes and Thespians) and Live Theater and it all began in high school and remained as a thread throughout her life.

Interview of an elderly person age 75-84 year of age

Harley Davidson (Pseudonym)

Question 1. Age 84

Question 2. As you look over your lifetime what is the one thing that makes you proud; My kids

Question 3. What is your future goal?

To be a financially successful author.

Question 4. If you could give advice to the younger generation what would it be?

Follow your bliss.

Question 5. What is the major change you've seen in our world in your lifetime and has it been a good one or a bad one?

Computers. Dangerous for loss of privacy and vulnerability to MWP attack

Question 6. Is there anything you would do differently if you had it to do over again?

I'd ask for SS credit for my work as a spy.

Question 7. What is the major challenge that you are facing now that you didn't have to deal with when you were younger?

My wife's disability.

Question 8. What is the one thing you enjoy doing?

Writing books

Question 9. What is the one thing that I didn't ask you about that you want to tell me or want the other students to know? No

Interview of an elderly person age 85+ year of age

Petticoat Junction Trixie (Pseudonym)

Question 1. Age? 88 yrs.

Question 2. As you look over your lifetime what is the one thing that makes you proud? She raised five kids and none of them are in jail. She lost her oldest daughter to cancer. She was 20 when she had her.

Question 3. What is your future goal? She wants to continue to live alone and she has a corgi puppy and she has a whole roll of tomato plants that she enjoys taking care of.

Question 4. If you could give advice to the younger generation what would it be? Set a goal and try to achieve it. You almost have to have a purpose in life or something that you are aiming for.

Question 5. What is the major change you've seen in our world in your lifetime and has it been a good one or a bad one? There has been a lot of improvement. She used to have to use the iron from an iron stove, they didn't have a refrigerator, they only had a well that they hung their milk jug in to keep it cold for supper, and they had no lights except Aladdin lamps. They had telephone lines but no electricity. But they didn't have a telephone either. Then they got electricity it as called REA electricity.

Question 6. Is there anything you would do differently if you had it to do over again? She doesn't hardly think so. Her daughter was an RN and she got her degree in Springfield. Her oldest son was a pianist but she wished he would have got in little band.

Question 7. What is the major challenge that you are facing now that you didn't have to deal with when you were younger? Eyesight

Question 8. What is the one thing you enjoy doing? She likes to dance, she likes to grow her tomatoes, she loves her Corgi doggie and she likes to give out food samples where she works.

Question 9. What is the one thing that I didn't ask you about that you want to tell me or want the other students to know? Her dad had milk cows and her husband had milk cows. They grew hay and had chickens. She taught school for two years in country schools grades one through eight.

Reflections of the Interview with Sweet Violet

I am only friends with the person I interviewed. She came up and introduced herself to me one day when I was doing some volunteer work at a recent entertainment function and we became friends after that because I realized we shared some very important views and values relating to entertainment.

We only met recently and have only been around each other for a few days. We have spoken a few times on the phone as well and gone out to lunch together. And I've taken her shopping a few times and to run some of her errands because she doesn't have a car. 1 John 3:17 "But whoso hath this world's good, and seeth his brother has need, and shutteth up his bowels of compassion from him, how dwelleth the love of God in him?" (1 John 3:17 King James Version).

I admire the way that she brags about her grandchildren. I also admire the way she gets to travel and stay in luxurious resorts all over with her time share packages. And that she gets to enjoy thousands of dollars on entertainment packages doing nothing but enjoying herself and eating the finest of foods, wearing the finest of clothing and jewelry. And most of all I admire her free-spirited independence.

She later told me that she was married though she was traveling alone and I know that marital transitions like travelling alone occur later in life for married couples (Ferrini, 2013 p. 198). And I learned that she has great independence even though she is very old. However, she is also blessed to have family support when she needs it too.

References: Ferrini, R., & Ferrini, A. (2013). The Study of Health and Aging. In *Health in the Later Years* (Fifth edition ed., pg. 198). New York: McGraw-Hill.

Personal Reflection

Some of them had unrealistic goals and not so honest answers to the questions. Sadly, I believe they did this as a self-protective measure due to their extreme physical and financial limitations.

Others had very realist goals according to their personal lifestyle that they were already exhibiting such as travel and leisure time spent with their family.

I can see where some of them need much more monetary and physical support as caregivers of their aging and disabled spouse because they are very old themselves and are having to care for a disabled senior citizen spouse with limited help and finances.

My suggestions would be that Medicare acknowledge and address this issue either through social programs or through private insurances companies.

Conclusion and Personal Perceptions on Aging

I have a great bit more respect for the elderly now. It is encouraging to know that we have such strong, loving citizens in our country and to know they are the backbone that this nation is built on.

I believe children need to have much more respect for their aging parents than what has been given to many of the elderly in the past.

There should be more programs like in home care services or maid and nursing services, transportation services, and more dental programs to fit the needs of those on Medicare.

More programs should be put in place to ensure that seniors have as much independence and support as needed to maintain a life of independence and integrity especially since the aging population is growing in our nation.

There should also be more programs in our society that would accommodate and include senior citizens.

Programs such as senior neighborhood programs and social events like Bridge or Bingo, community lunches or dinners should be implemented in every community.

They should provide services, events and things that they could all participate in because many senior citizens do not have family or friends that they can rely on for support or for companions. Aging is a very vulnerable part of life and it should be protected for all.

The AARP www.aarp.org has a lot of programs that are geared to help senior citizens get discounts and affordable necessities too.

Belief Statement

Kimmy Gerred

Abstract

Purpose: To declare my belief and philosophy concerning the elderly, seniors, and retired persons.

Methods: Observe my life in relation to the seniors that are part of my life now and how the bible effects my relationships to the seniors.

Results: There are a few seniors in my life that I relate to specifically to help them reach their goals of living *independent and it enables me to be a part of the pure gospel by including them in my life.*

Conclusion: *Taking care of the elderly is a ministry because of the verse in James 1:27. And it is also helping society by helping seniors, elderly and retired to stay active in their relations and hopefully active with their lifestyle which both have shown to prolong health, independence and longer life.*

Key Words and Tags: Prevention Research, Elderly, seniors, Aging, Senior Citizens, Retired, Nursing

Homes, Long-term care, Adult Daycare

Belief Statement

My Philosophy

I believe that when one begins to age, they begin a distinct emptying of themselves and there is not much of a way to prevent it. I also believe that some of the greatest and wisest souls on earth can only be found in the elderly, seniors and retired people. Not only are they important for their contributions to society but God says they are of utmost importance in James 1:27 "Pure religion and undefiled before God and the Father is this, To visit the fatherless and widows in their affliction, and to keep himself unspotted from the world." (James 1:27 King James Version). Scripture also says it like this "The silver-haired head is a crown of glory, if it is found in the way of righteousness."

(Proverbs 16:31)

Worldview of the Elderly

I believe that we are to watch over, guard and protect all who are weak including the elderly, seniors and retired. We are to try and make things easier for the elderly, seniors and the retired. If they have to do a difficult task I believe that the younger healthier people in the community of the church or family should be there at every turn to help them achieve the task for them or with them.

The scripture also says that pure religion is to take care of the orphans, the widows and the weak. "Pure religion and undefiled before God and the Father is this, to visit the fatherless and widows in their affliction, and to keep himself unspotted from the world." (James 1:27 King James Version)

Elderly Persons in My Life

There are about nine elderly people in my life. Three of them are like family and they are very far away so they are unable to be a regular part of my life. The rest are friends who live nearby of which a few of them converse with me on a weekly basis. Another one who I was fairly close to has been taken to a private care facility and her power of attorney has refused to allow her to see or talk to me and another one of her friends, so she is really no longer able to be an active part of my life as I wish she could be. Two of the seniors I have over on regular basis for Holiday get together and celebratory feasts like the Passover meal. And two more of the seniors in my life are active in my life for going on outings to the grocery store and other places in our community.

All of these people are very important to me and because we live in an extreme environment If I am not able to reach them by phone or any other way I have relied on the police department to go and check on them. Thankfully, the police department have been very cooperative with me to go and check on a very frail elderly person when I could not reach them by phone or any other way. They are more than friends, I count some of them as close friends or parental figures in my life.

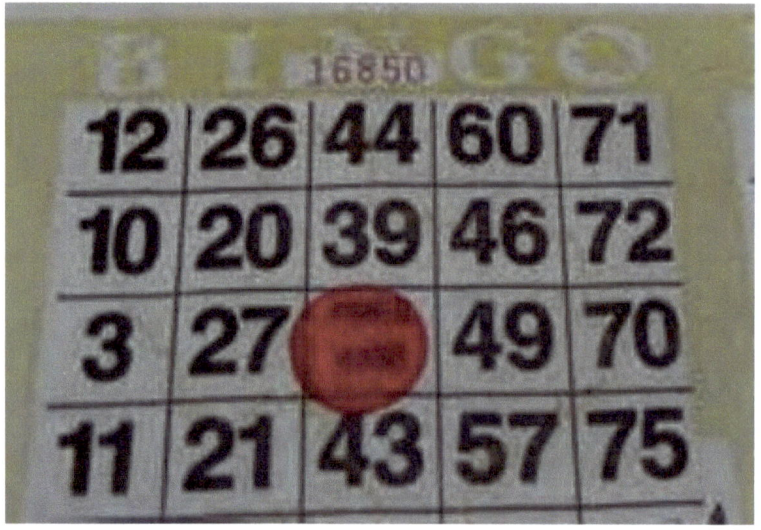

Health Promotion as a Ministry

Health Promotion can be a ministry if you ask a senior to join you for a lap at the pool, or for a walk in the park. That is your time that you are investing in caring for the needs of someone else. And that is the pure gospel and undefiled religion when we spend time with seniors, elderly and retired as it says in James 1:27.

I consider working with the elderly a great privilege that God has bestowed upon me because they have so much that I can glean from. I love to listen to their wisdom, their beliefs and learn from their way of doing. To me, it is like taking a learning skill or trade when I get to glean from their lives.

My Ministry Contributions to the Elderly & Their Contributions

I can give my elderly friends rides to the store or to run their errands. I also cook nice dinners for them and have them all over to commune and sup with me and we then enjoy each other's company. I learn information from the past first-hand. Information that no other can offer me and information that is unlikely to be found in any books. To me, this is a great treasure! And to have their company is also of great value to me.

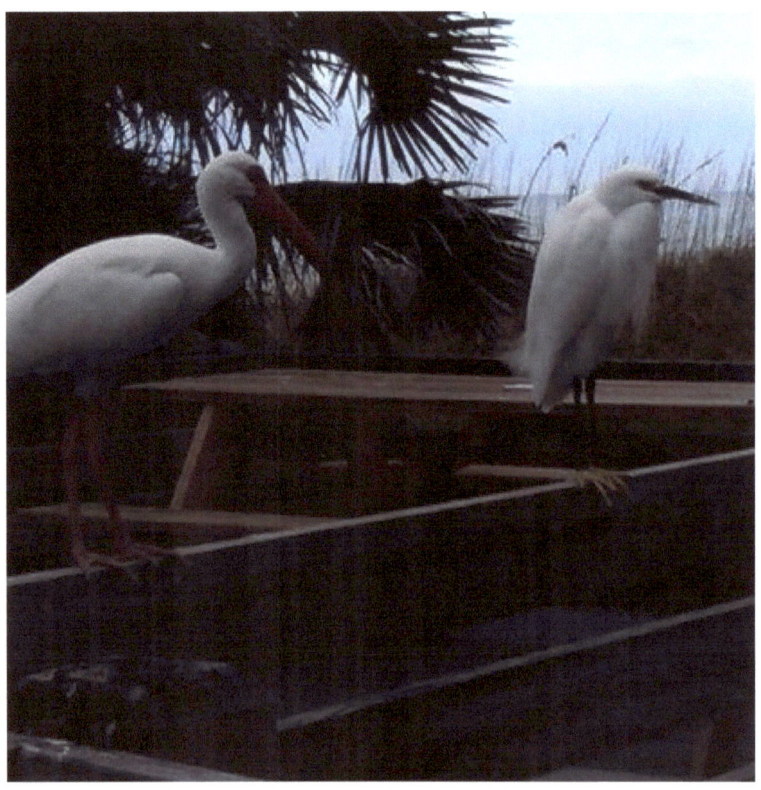

What I Can Do to Effect My Own Aging Process

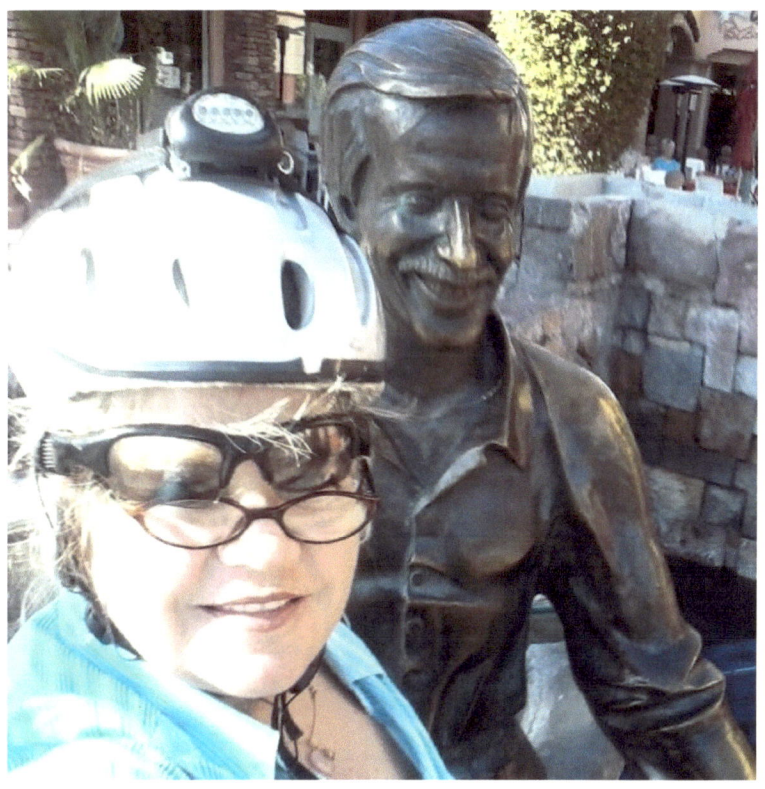

I began eating more healthy foods, removing the not so healthy foods out of my grocery list. I found that if I don't buy them then I cannot use them to cook with or to eat them. I am hoping that my changed diet will help me progress towards a healthy body day by day, week by week, month by month and year by year. Sometimes it takes time to undo the bad that has been done.

And sometimes it takes time for the new ways to show the benefits of the change. I need to exercise but the pain of the arthritis is so debilitating that I have to take pain medicines and anti-inflammatory medicine just to be able to ride my bike which is the only land exercise that my physical therapists have approved for me.

Now that I know that the sedentary lifestyle is the one that causes disability to worsen, and sedentary lifestyle also prohibits people from recovering from injuries or illness, and sedentary lifestyle also shortens life spans I will fight the pain harder to keep myself active 4 times per week from now on beginning now. If I ride my bike or do laps in the pool then that will be enough to interrupt the sedentary lifestyle that I have lived for much of the past decade.

  I am already over the age of fifty and I've worked very hard on my health by quitting smoking, I don't live a risky lifestyle of sexual impurity or alcohol consumption so the only thing I need to do is to add exercise and continue the other healthy choices that I have made then I can see myself at age seventy in better health than I was at age fifty.

My Perceptions of Working with the Elderly

My parents are gone already so a few of these seniors I kind of relate to as the senior authority in my life and I honor them as that. I watch out for them and try to assist them in any ways that I can like I would have done for my parents if they were still alive. I consider it a privilege and a responsibility to have seniors, retired persons and the elderly in my life. I think it is a great reference to have for future prospects of positions in the work force.

My Future Life When I am 70 Year of Age

I see myself still writing and publishing books, still being an activist with the gospel of Christ Jesus and doing whatever my hands find to do to the glory of God. Health and independence will be important to me at age seventy so I will do my part in working daily to achieve health and overcome the sedentary lifestyle.

References

> Ferrini & Ferrini (see p. 391, p. 99 The Study of Health and Aging Introduction)
>
> James 1:27 King James Version, Proverbs 16:31 King James Version

Helpful tips and useful information

"Epidemiologists report that the greatest impact on chronic illness can be made through lifestyle changes rather than technological interventions such as drugs or surgery." (Ferrini & Ferrini pg.391)

A sedentary lifestyle is associated with many debilitating and life-threatening diseases including heart disease, hypertension, obesity, osteoporosis, diabetes, and mental disorders. It has also been associated with shorter life spans and reduced ability to recover from injuries or illness.

Exercise is used in prevention, treatment and control of high blood pressure. Exercise is also associated with lower risk of early death.

Physical Fitness and Fall Prevention

Balance, endurance, strengthening and flexibility are all important for good health.

Balance exercises can be done by placing your hand on a wall or a chair and doing side and back leg lifts. Also by standing on one foot and by walking heel to toe.

Ten to Fifteen (10-15) repetitions of leg lifts then slowly increase the challenge by removing the chair or the wall to balance.

Endurance can be done by swimming, walking, gardening, raking, or cycling 30 minutes per day five days a week.

Strengthening can be done by free weights or squeeze balls and can prevent falling and maintain functioning through life. Lift a can of soup or a free weight and squeeze a ball two (2) or more days a week for thirty (30) minutes each time. Start light with elastic bands and you can do 8-12 repetitions for (3) seconds lift or push and hold for one (1) second then release or return for (3) seconds.

Flexibility can be done by stretching all muscle groups before any exercise. Stretch 3-5 times each session hold for 10-30 second while doing it slow and smooth stretches, breath deep and stretch farther each time.

Doing these exercises will help you to maintain physical activity. Think of the ole saying "use it or lose it" to describe the importance of exercise.

Some Useful Links For Seniors

www.thewalkingsite.com

Two More Golden Rules For Seniors

Immunize and take a daily aspirin are primary prevention steps that older people need to take.

www.ahrq.gov Agency for Health Care Research and Quality www.cdc Centers for Disease Control www.aoa.dhhs.gov Administration on Aging www.nia.hih.gov National Institute on Aging www.healthypeople.gov
www.uspreventiveservicestaskforc.org/adultrec.htm
www.asaging.org American Society on Aging
www.med-decisions.com

Immunizations
Influenza

Pneumonia

Hepatitis B

Screening services
Glaucoma

Nutrition therapy

Cervical cancer

Pelvic exam

Breast cancer

Osteoporosis (Bone mass densitometry)

Colon cancer

Diabetes

Prostate cancer

"Welcome to Medicare" exam

Cholesterol screening

Human Immunodeficiency Virus (HIV)

Tobacco counseling

Abdominal aortic aneurysm screening

Yearly wellness visit

Alcohol Use Information

The use of "alcohol provokes the desire but takes away sexual performance" is well documented. Blood alcohol levels may accelerate sexual arousal by reducing inhibitions, but it also diminishes performance. It also causes reduced blood supply to the organs, reduces testosterone levels and testicular size. It reduces nerve sensitivity in the male sexual organ (word omitted on purpose) and has negative effect on the ability to achieve and maintain an erection. It causes temporary erectile dysfunction and can cause irreversible loss of erectile function even if drinking is stopped. (Ferrini & Ferrini pg. 361)

Medicare Nursing Home Compare

Kimmy Gerred

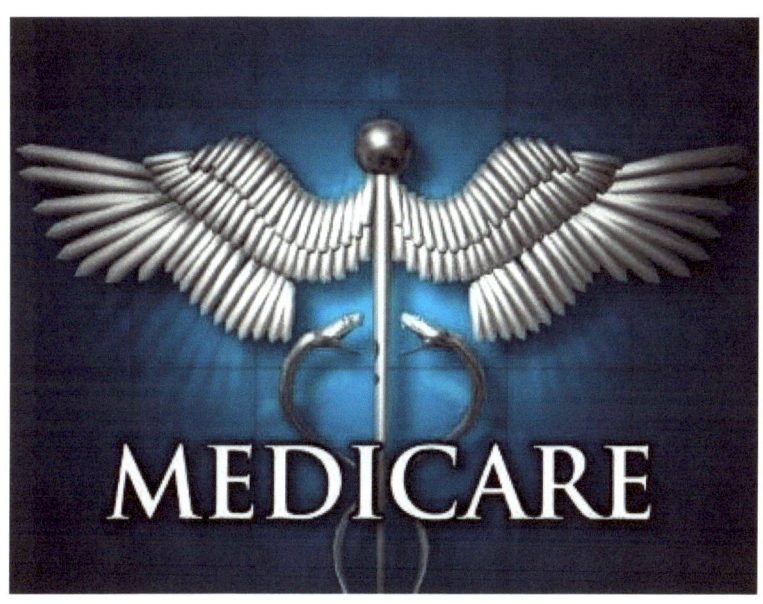

Abstract

Medicare Nursing Home Compare Purpose: To know how a nursing home adds up or compares to other nursing homes in the vicinity. To learn if there have been any penalties for that particular nursing home. To research a nursing home to see if it is suitable for your loved ones needs.

Medicare Nursing Home Compare Methods:

Go to www.medicare.gov/nursinghomecompare and put in the zip code of the facility we are researching. Then chose the name of the facility from the list that pops up and click on it. Then begin by clicking the tabs which have the information in which we were searching and read the data and details there.

Nursing Home Reflections: The nursing home seemed to be a bit more above average than what the Medicare.gov website rated it. That maybe because I've been in about four other nursing homes and the one that I researched smelled better than them all.

Conclusion: I am glad that nursing homes are available for our dear senior friends who need an extra hand in caring for themselves and for living a healthy life. If either of my parents were alive I would do all I could do within my power to make sure that they didn't have to live in a nursing home.

Key Words and Tags: Prevention Research, Elderly, Nursing Homes, Long-term Care, Adult daycare, Aging, Senior Citizens

Medicare Nursing Home Compare

Overall Mountain Springs Healthcare & Rehabilitation Center (Name Changed to protect the privacy) only scored average on their "overall" rating or three (3) stars. However, in "quality measures" they scored above average with four (4) stars.

MEDIGAP BENEFITS	MEDIGAP PLANS									
	A	B	C	D	F	G	K	L	M	N
Medicare Part A Coinsurance and hospital costs up to an additional 365 days after Medicare benefits are used up	√	√	√	√	√	√	√	√	√	√
Medicare Part B Coinsurance or Copayment	√	√	√	√	√	√	50%	75%	√	√
Blood (First 3 Pints)	√	√	√	√	√	√	50%	75%	√	√
Part A Hospice Care Coinsurance or Copayment	√	√	√	√	√	√	50%	75%	√	√
Skilled Nursing Facility Care Coinsurance			√	√	√	√	50%	75%	√	√
Medicare Part A Deductible		√	√	√	√	√	50%	75%	50%	√
Medicare Part B Deductible			√		√					
Medicare Part B Excess Charges					√	√				
Foreign Travel Emergency (Up to Plan Limits)			√	√	√	√			√	√

Every time that I was ever there, I thought that it was cleaner than other nursing homes that I had visited. I learned that they have never had any penalties in the last three (3) years. And that they have a sprinkler system.

I have considered working in a nursing home and I have worked with some churches in Clearwater to go and visit the elderly. At that time I don't recall it being so difficult for me to handle as it is now. Now, I am a bit more reserved at being around older people than I was fifteen years ago. I have a tendency to absorb whatever I'm around and with my current health issues that is why I guess I am a bit more reserved about being around them on a constant everyday basis.

But because of my health issues and my moral values most all of my friends are over the age of retirement or could be considered retired with only a few exceptions. I've thought about this and asked myself how could this be? And the only thing that my senior friends have in common with my younger friends is that none of them drink alcohol around me, none of them smoke, and none of them use drugs, or participate in sexual immorality.

In the area of California where I live it is particularly difficult to find such kind of people who are my age or younger but I do have one friend like that. He is actually younger than me by five years. I'm grateful for all my friends though the rest of them (about five) are all over ten years older than me.

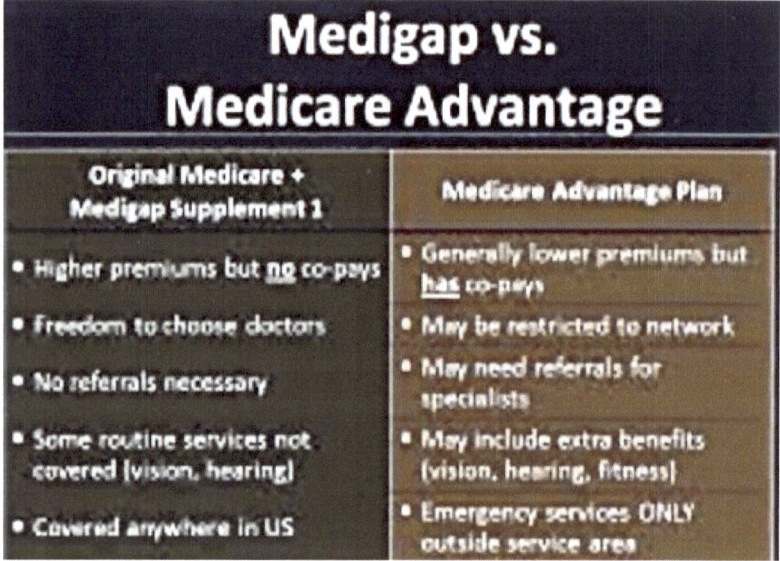

But only one of them I hang out with and have in my car without any reserves because she is well groomed and in very strong and mobile health. Some old people have a distinct "old person" smell and because of my health issues I've learned what causes that smell is from not washing your hair on a daily basis. It gathers oil and follicle dander and produces that strange 'old person smell' I try to consider that now when grooming my hair. Because there are salon oils and hair conditioners that can remedy that.

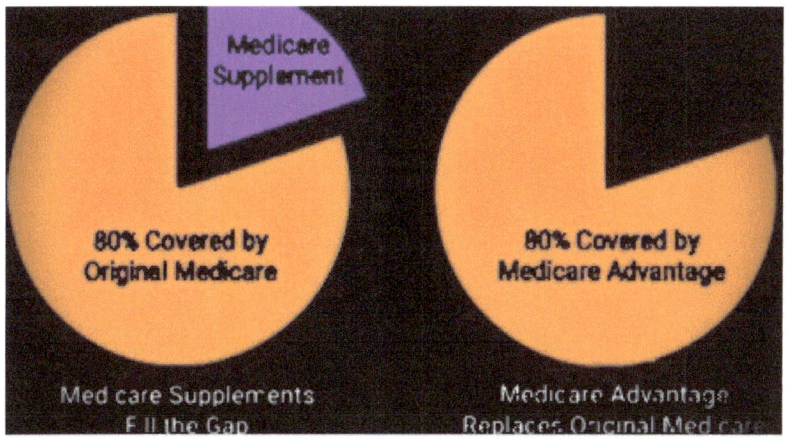

It also bothers me a bit about the stats on nursing home sexual and physical abuse. I almost develop this mentality that looks at men nurses with a "ah, I know what you did" mind frameset. Particularly if they are large men or domineering men. And I also look at patients and wonder what have they suffered in silence and it breaks my heart.

An important fact to remember is "Epidemiologists report the greatest impact on chronic illness can be made through lifestyle changes rather than technological interventions such as drugs or surgery.' (Ferrini & Ferrini page 391)

But then again, it is very hard for some who are dealing with mobility challenges to push past their pain of arthritis to do the necessary exercises to improve their overall health. That is when we must remember that all life is God's gift to mankind and we need to be kind and compassionate to those who have already given of themselves in this lifetime and now they need others to give back to them. Matthew 25:40 KJV "And the King shall answer and say unto them, Verily I say unto you, Inasmuch as ye have done it unto one of the least of these my brethren, ye have done it unto me." (Matthew 25:40 King James Version)

I'm thankful that my mother lived at home with her husband until they admitted her into the hospital where she later died. Knowing what I know now, I would not put my loved one in a nursing home unless I absolutely could not care for them myself. I know that they are probably not as bad as they appear to be. And that God is in control even of what goes on at Nursing homes. It is just so sad to also know that some suffering has also happened to some of the patients who resided at nursing homes.

References

Ferrini & Ferrini (pg. 391 The Study Of Health and Aging Introduction)

Matthew 25:40 King James Version

Medicare.Gov/nursinghomecompare Nursing Home Compare

Futures for The Elderly

Kimmy Gerred

"60 million people are expected to have #Alzheimer's #disease by 2040." http://www.alzinfo.org/http://www.alzinfo.org/ (Frederick Serriere @FredSerriere on Twitter)

"25 million adult American's experience transient or chronic urinary incontinence." The exercise that can remedy both Stress incontinence of urinary and fecal incontinence is the Kegel exercises.

Stress incontinence occurs when a person sneezes, coughs, jumping or laughing to hard putting extra pressure on a full bladder triggering the bladder to leak urine.

The elderly should be able to keep their dignity and have all of their personal morals respected. I believe they should be able to have access to all of their family and friends that they were accustomed to speaking with or seeing on a regular basis even if they are put in a private care facility.

Kegel exercise is done by tightening the pelvic floor muscles. A person can sit on the toilet and begin to urinate, then try to stop the flow by tightening the muscles in the pelvic floor but the abdomen, thigh or buttocks should not be affected.

Tighten the pelvic floor muscles and hold for the count of ten then release it completely and count to ten. Do these ten times in the morning, afternoon and bedtime or three times a day. Some experience improvement in three weeks, others in three months.

I do not believe that seniors or elderly should ever be deprived access to their friends or family. If they don't like to be around cussing or watch television programs with immoral activity on it then they should not be subject to change their morals once they are put in a private care family.

My friend was taken into a private care facility in August of last year. They denied her access to speak to me or to our other mutual friend. When we would go to visit her, they would tell us that it was forbidden. When we would call they also forbid her to speak on the phone unless we went through a lady who forcefully took the power of attorney from our friend.

Recently a "Ghost Boy" awoke from a 12-year coma. Doctors told his parents and caregivers that he did not know or understand anything that was happening around him or if anyone spoke to him.

When he awoke from the coma, he told everyone that he saw and knew everything going on around him. He tells how he saw sexual and physical abuse at every single nursing home or in home private care sitter's facility that he was placed in. And that it was only by chance that he didn't get molested at one of the places he was put in. See the video on "[Thomas Nelson's](...)" YouTube channel here http://youtu.be/1CIybH86gP0

I don't think America respects the elderly the way that the elderly deserves to be respected. 1 Timothy 5 says we are to care for the elderly and give them honor and respect. 1 Timothy 5:1 "Do not rebuke an older man harshly but exhort him as if he were your father."

I don't think people realize how important it is for our elderly to be checked on, visited loved and respected. I think it is important to realize that the elderly person could be one step from eternity where their soul destination will be eternally decided for better or worse.

I think that society needs to realize that the elderly is some of society's most vulnerable and most important because their soul destination could be determined in the very last days they have here on earth and Long-Term Care facilities need to be aware of that and make plenty of provision for the elderly's spiritual needs as well as their physical needs by providing them some physical exercise that they can do safely, some mental exercises that they can do socially so they can make connections and remain active with their relationships and thoughts during their last years on earth.

Robert Louis Stevenson says it like this "Old and young, we are all on our last cruise. Ferrini & Ferrini (see p. 1 The Study of Health and Aging Introduction)

Find more resources

At https://cainsure.blogspot.com

Or at www.cahealthinsure.blogspot.com

Also, find Kimmy On Facebook at
https://www.facebook.com/InsureCalifornia/

Since the original publication of this book, my dear friend Dr. Hans J. Petermann who was interviewed in this book passed away on August 03, 2016. He was my favorite Thanksgiving Day guest. Just a few weeks before he passed away our mutual friend (his lady friend) that I like to think of as his love light told me something, he said about me to her.

It was the 2nd nicest compliment that I've ever had in my life. First being when my daughter told me that she wouldn't feel comfortable letting anyone else babysit her first born child (my gran- daughter) while she was away at the hospital giving birth to her sisters. She said I was the only one she trusted to take care of her. That was the greatest compliment a grandmother could ever have!

Dr. Hans told our female friend

"Kimmy gave me the most meaningful gift of sharing like-minded intelligence. She is dynamic and inspirational and gave me strength to finish my book. She means so much to me and has helped me intellectually and personally. She is my closest friend here and I spend Thanksgivings with her as her cooking is delicious."

I only knew that he felt this way about me a few weeks before he passed away. She told me that he thought that I was the greatest thing on earth. That blew my mind as I had no idea!! He is still so very missed!

www.ingramcontent.com/pod-product-compliance
Lightning Source LLC
Chambersburg PA
CBHW040224220526
45473CB00001B/111